THE IBS DIET BIBLE

A Beginner's Guide To Managing IBS With Delicious, Healthful Recipes And Meal Plans

CRUE GAGE

Table of Contents

Introductory

Irritable Bowel Syndrome (IBS) is a prevalent gastrointestinal disorder that impacts the large intestine. It is distinguished by a variety of symptoms, such as abdominal pain, bloating, flatulence, diarrhea, and constipation. The precise cause of IBS is not well understood; however,

it may be a combination of abnormal gut motility, gut-brain interaction, and sensitivity to specific foods or stress. Certain foods, stress, hormonal changes, and other factors can induce symptoms that can vary significantly among individuals. Lifestyle and dietary modifications, stress management, and occasionally medication are frequently implemented during treatment.

Common symptoms of Irritable Bowel Syndrome (IBS) include:

- **Abdominal Pain or Cramping**: Often relieved by bowel movements.

- **Bloating**: A feeling of fullness or swelling in the abdomen.

- **Gas**: Increased flatulence or belching.

- **Diarrhea**: Frequent loose or watery stools.

- **Constipation**: Infrequent or difficult bowel movements.

- **Alternating Symptoms**: Some people experience a mix of diarrhea and constipation.

<u>**Common triggers can include:**</u>

- **Certain Foods**: High-fat foods, dairy products, caffeine, artificial sweeteners, and spicy foods.

- **Stress**: Emotional or psychological stress can worsen symptoms.

- **Hormonal Changes**: Symptoms may fluctuate with menstrual cycles in women.

- **Gut Infections**: Previous gastrointestinal infections can trigger IBS in some individuals.

- **Lifestyle Factors**: Lack of physical activity, irregular eating patterns, and insufficient sleep may contribute.

Identifying personal triggers can be helpful for managing symptoms.

CHAPTER ONE
How Food Affects Ibs Symptoms

Food can have a significant impact on IBS symptoms. Different foods may trigger or worsen symptoms for different individuals. Here are some key ways food affects IBS:

• **Trigger Foods**: Common triggers include high-fat foods, dairy products, caffeine, spicy foods, and foods containing artificial sweeteners. Keeping a food diary can help identify personal triggers.

• **FODMAPs**: Some people with IBS are sensitive to fermentable oligosaccharides, disaccharides, monosaccharides, and polyols (FODMAPs). These are types of carbohydrates that can lead to gas and bloating. A low-FODMAP diet, which reduces these foods, can be beneficial.

• **Fiber Intake**: Fiber can be beneficial, but the type matters. Soluble fiber (found in oats, fruits, and vegetables) may help with constipation, while insoluble fiber (found in whole grains and some vegetables) can exacerbate symptoms for some individuals.

• **Eating Patterns**: Irregular eating habits, such as skipping meals or overeating, can trigger symptoms. Regular, balanced meals are generally recommended.

• **Hydration**: Staying hydrated is important, especially for those experiencing constipation. Drinking enough water can help with digestion.

• **Alcohol and Caffeine**: These can irritate the gut and may worsen symptoms for some individuals.

Managing diet carefully can lead to better symptom control for many people with IBS.

The Importance Of Personalized Nutrition

Personalized nutrition is crucial, especially for conditions like Irritable Bowel Syndrome (IBS), because each individual reacts differently to foods. Here's why it matters:

• **Unique Responses**: People have varying sensitivities to certain foods and ingredients. What triggers symptoms in one person may be well-tolerated by another.

• **Identifying Triggers**: Personalized nutrition helps individuals identify specific food triggers through methods like food diaries or elimination diets, leading to tailored dietary choices.

• **Enhanced Symptom Management**: By focusing on foods that soothe rather than irritate the gut, individuals can better manage symptoms and improve their quality of life.

• **Nutritional Balance**: A personalized approach ensures that individuals still receive essential nutrients while avoiding foods that cause discomfort.

• **Behavioral and Lifestyle Factors**: Personalizing nutrition also takes into account lifestyle factors, such as stress management, physical activity, and eating habits, all of which can influence gut health.

- **Long-Term Success**: A tailored nutrition plan is more sustainable and effective in the long run, as it aligns with individual preferences and lifestyles.

Personalized nutrition allows for a more effective and individualized approach to managing IBS and other dietary-related conditions, enhancing overall health and well-being.

The exact cause of Irritable Bowel Syndrome (IBS) is not fully understood, but several factors may contribute to its development:

<u>Causes:</u>

• **Gut-Brain Interaction**: Dysfunction in the communication between the brain and gut can lead to altered gut motility and sensitivity.

• **Abnormal Gut Motility**: Changes in the speed of digestion can cause symptoms like diarrhea or constipation.

• **Intestinal Inflammation**: Some people report a history of gastrointestinal infections that can trigger IBS.

• **Microbiome Imbalance**: Changes in the gut bacteria (microbiome) may play a role in IBS development.

• **Food Sensitivities**: Certain foods may exacerbate symptoms, particularly those high in FODMAPs.

<u>Risk Factors:</u>

• **Age**: IBS can occur at any age but is more common in younger adults.

• **Gender**: Women are more likely to be diagnosed with IBS than men, possibly due to hormonal factors.

• **Family History**: A family history of IBS or other gastrointestinal disorders may increase risk.

• **Mental Health**: Conditions like anxiety and depression are linked to IBS and can influence symptom severity.

• **Previous Gastrointestinal Infections**: A history of infections can increase the likelihood of developing IBS.

• **Stress**: High levels of stress or traumatic life events may trigger or worsen symptoms.

Understanding these causes and risk factors can help in identifying potential triggers and developing effective management strategies for IBS.

Prevention & Treatment Options

Preventing and managing Irritable Bowel Syndrome (IBS) involves a combination of lifestyle changes, dietary adjustments, and medical interventions. Here are some options:

Prevention:

• **Dietary Management**: Identifying and avoiding trigger foods can help prevent symptom flare-ups. Keeping a food diary can be useful.

• **Regular Exercise**: Engaging in regular physical activity can help improve gut motility and reduce stress.

• **Stress Management**: Techniques such as mindfulness, yoga, and relaxation exercises can help manage stress, which may trigger symptoms.

• **Adequate Sleep**: Ensuring good sleep hygiene can contribute to overall gut health and symptom management.

Dietary Changes:

- **Low-FODMAP Diet**: This involves reducing high-FODMAP foods to alleviate symptoms.
- **Increase Soluble Fiber**: Foods high in soluble fiber (like oats and fruits) can help with constipation.

Medications:

- **Antispasmodics**: Help relieve abdominal cramping and pain.
- **Laxatives**: For those experiencing constipation.
- **Antidiarrheal Medications**: For diarrhea-predominant IBS.
- **Prescription Medications**: Such as linaclotide or lubiprostone for constipation-predominant IBS, and

rifaximin for diarrhea-predominant IBS.

Psychological Therapies:

- **Cognitive Behavioral Therapy (CBT)**: Can help address anxiety and stress related to IBS.

- **Gut-Directed Hypnotherapy**: Some find relief through guided relaxation and visualization techniques.

- **Probiotics**: Some studies suggest that probiotics may help improve gut health and alleviate symptoms for certain individuals.

- **Lifestyle Modifications**: Regular meal schedules, adequate hydration, and mindful eating practices can contribute to symptom management.

It's important for individuals to work closely with healthcare providers to tailor prevention and treatment strategies to their specific needs and symptoms.

CHAPTER TWO
What Are FODMAPs?

FODMAPs are a group of fermentable carbohydrates that can be poorly absorbed in the small intestine, leading to digestive issues for some individuals, particularly those with Irritable Bowel Syndrome (IBS). The acronym stands for:

- **Fermentable**: These carbohydrates can be fermented by gut bacteria, producing gas.

- **Oligosaccharides**: Found in foods like wheat, onions, and garlic.

- **Disaccharides**: Primarily lactose, found in dairy products like milk and soft cheese.

- **Monosaccharides**: Fructose, found in honey, apples, and high-fructose corn syrup.

- **Polyols**: Sugar alcohols like sorbitol and mannitol, found in some fruits and artificial sweeteners.

For people sensitive to FODMAPs, consuming these foods can lead to symptoms like bloating, gas, abdominal pain, diarrhea, and constipation. The low-FODMAP diet involves reducing these foods and gradually reintroducing them to identify specific triggers.

Foods To Avoid & Foods To Include

Here's a breakdown of foods to avoid and include when following a low-FODMAP dict:

Foods to Avoid (High-FODMAP):

Oligosaccharides:

- Wheat products (bread, pasta)

- Onions and garlic

- Legumes (beans, lentils, chickpeas)

Disaccharides:

• Dairy products high in lactose (milk, soft cheeses, yogurt)

Monosaccharides:

- High-fructose fruits (apples, pears, cherries)

- Honey and high-fructose corn syrup

Polyols:

- Certain fruits (avocado, cherries, plums)

- Sugar alcohols (sorbitol, mannitol, found in sugar-free products)

- Foods to Include (Low-FODMAP):

Grains:

- Rice, oats, quinoa, gluten-free grains (corn, millet)

Fruits:

- Bananas, blueberries, strawberries, oranges, grapes

Vegetables:

- Carrots, spinach, zucchini, bell peppers, cucumbers

Proteins:

- Meat, poultry, fish, eggs, tofu (firm)

Dairy Alternatives:

- Lactose-free milk and yogurt
- Hard cheeses (cheddar, parmesan)

Nuts and Seeds:

• Almonds (in moderation), walnuts, pumpkin seeds

Oils and Fats:

• Olive oil, coconut oil, butter (in moderation)

Always consult a healthcare provider or dietitian before starting a low-FODMAP diet to ensure it's done safely and effectively. After a period of restriction, foods can be gradually reintroduced to identify personal triggers.

Identifying Trigger Foods & How To Conduct An Elimination Diet

Identifying trigger foods and conducting an elimination diet can be effective for managing IBS symptoms. Here's a guide on how to do it:

Identifying Trigger Foods:

- **Keep a Food Diary**: Track everything you eat and drink, along with symptoms, timing, and severity. This helps identify patterns and potential triggers.

- **Look for Common Triggers**: Note if symptoms consistently follow certain foods or meals, especially high-FODMAP foods.

- **Assess Portion Sizes**: Sometimes, smaller amounts of a trigger food may be tolerated, so consider portion sizes in your diary.

Conducting an Elimination Diet:

- **Choose a Timeframe**: Typically, an elimination phase lasts 4-6 weeks. This allows time to see if symptoms improve.

- **Eliminate High-FODMAP Foods**: Remove high-FODMAP foods identified from your diary and general lists from your diet during this period.

- **Plan Balanced Meals**: Ensure you're still getting adequate nutrition by including low-FODMAP foods across all food groups.

- **Monitor Symptoms**: Keep tracking symptoms throughout the elimination phase to determine if they improve.

- **Reintroduction Phase**: After the elimination phase, reintroduce high-FODMAP foods one at a time every few days. This helps identify specific triggers.

- Start with small amounts and gradually increase the portion.

- Monitor and record any symptoms that occur after reintroduction.

After the reintroduction phase, review your food diary to see which foods triggered symptoms and adjust your diet accordingly.

Important Considerations:

- **Consult a Professional**: It's advisable to work with a registered dietitian or healthcare provider when conducting an elimination diet to ensure it's done safely and nutritionally balanced.

- **Be Patient**: Identifying triggers can take time and may require several cycles of elimination and reintroduction.

7 Days Sample Meal Plans

Here's a 7-day sample meal plan for a low-FODMAP diet. Adjust portion sizes based on individual needs and preferences.

Day 1:

- **Breakfast**: Oatmeal made with lactose-free milk, topped with blueberries.
- **Snack**: A banana.

- **Lunch**: Grilled chicken salad with spinach, cucumbers, and a lemon-olive oil dressing.
- **Snack**: Rice cakes with peanut butter.
- **Dinner**: Baked salmon with quinoa and steamed zucchini.

Day 2:

- **Breakfast**: Scrambled eggs with spinach and tomatoes.
- **Snack**: Orange slices.
- **Lunch**: Quinoa salad with bell peppers, carrots, and a vinaigrette.
- **Snack**: Lactose-free yogurt with strawberries.
- **Dinner**: Grilled shrimp with rice and sautéed green beans.

Day 3:

- **Breakfast**: Smoothie with lactose-free yogurt, spinach, and strawberries.
- **Snack**: A kiwi.
- **Lunch**: Turkey and lettuce wraps with sliced bell peppers.
- **Snack**: Almonds (in moderation).
- **Dinner**: Stir-fried chicken with bell peppers and carrots, served with rice.

Day 4:

- **Breakfast**: Rice cereal with lactose-free milk and sliced banana.
- **Snack**: Carrot sticks with hummus (check for low-FODMAP ingredients).

- **Lunch**: Grilled vegetable salad with mixed greens and a balsamic dressing.
- **Snack**: Popcorn (plain, no added butter).
- **Dinner**: Baked tilapia with mashed potatoes (made with lactose-free milk) and steamed broccoli.

Day 5:

- **Breakfast**: Chia pudding made with lactose-free milk and topped with strawberries.
- **Snack**: Sliced cucumber with a sprinkle of salt.
- **Lunch**: Chicken soup with low-FODMAP vegetables (like carrots and zucchini).

- **Snack**: Rice cakes with lactose-free cheese.
- **Dinner**: Beef stir-fry with broccoli and bell peppers, served over rice.

Day 6:

- **Breakfast**: Smoothie with lactose-free yogurt, spinach, and pineapple.
- **Snack**: Grapes.
- **Lunch**: Quinoa and roasted vegetable bowl with olive oil dressing.
- **Snack**: Hard-boiled egg.
- **Dinner**: Grilled pork chops with mashed sweet potatoes and sautéed spinach.

<u>Day 7:</u>

- **Breakfast**: Omelet with tomatoes and spinach.
- **Snack**: A small handful of walnuts.
- **Lunch**: Lentil soup (using low-FODMAP ingredients) with a side salad.
- **Snack**: Lactose-free yogurt with blueberries.
- **Dinner**: Roasted chicken with rice and steamed carrots.

<u>Tips:</u>

- Always check ingredient labels for potential high-FODMAP ingredients.
- Adjust meals based on personal preferences and tolerances.

- Consider hydration and aim for plenty of water throughout the week.

CHAPTER THREE
Breakfast Recipes

Here are some easy and delicious low-FODMAP breakfast recipes:

1. Oatmeal with Blueberries:

Ingredients:

- 1 cup rolled oats
- 2 cups lactose-free milk (or water)
- 1/2 cup blueberries
- A pinch of salt
- Maple syrup or brown sugar (optional)

Instructions:

- In a pot, combine oats, lactose-free milk, and a pinch of salt.
- Bring to a boil, then reduce heat and simmer for about 5 minutes, stirring occasionally.

- Remove from heat, stir in blueberries, and sweeten if desired.

2. *Scrambled Eggs with Spinach:*

Ingredients:

- 2 eggs
- A handful of fresh spinach
- Salt and pepper to taste
- 1 tsp olive oil or butter

Instructions:

- Heat olive oil or butter in a pan over medium heat.
- Add spinach and sauté until wilted.
- Whisk eggs in a bowl, season with salt and pepper, then pour into the pan.
- Stir gently until eggs are cooked to your liking.

3. Chia Pudding:

Ingredients:

- 1/4 cup chia seeds
- 1 cup lactose-free milk (or almond milk)
- 1 tsp maple syrup (optional)
- Fresh fruit (like strawberries or kiwi) for topping

Instructions:

- In a bowl or jar, combine chia seeds, lactose-free milk, and maple syrup.
- Stir well, then refrigerate for at least 4 hours or overnight.
- Serve topped with fresh fruit.

4. Smoothie Bowl:

Ingredients:

- 1 banana (ripe)
- 1/2 cup lactose-free yogurt
- 1/2 cup spinach
- 1/2 cup frozen strawberries
- Toppings: sliced kiwi, nuts, or seeds

Instructions:

- In a blender, combine banana, lactose-free yogurt, spinach, and frozen strawberries. Blend until smooth.
- Pour into a bowl and add your choice of toppings.

5. Rice Cereal with Banana:

Ingredients:

- 1 cup rice cereal (check for low-FODMAP)
- 1 cup lactose-free milk

- 1 banana, sliced

Instructions:

- In a bowl, combine rice cereal and lactose-free milk.
- Top with sliced banana and enjoy.

Feel free to mix and match ingredients based on your preferences and tolerances!

Lunch Recipes

<u>**Here are some tasty low-FODMAP lunch recipes:**</u>

1. Quinoa Salad with Grilled Chicken:

Ingredients:

- 1 cup cooked quinoa
- 1 grilled chicken breast, sliced
- 1 cup mixed greens (spinach, arugula)
- 1/2 cucumber, diced
- 1/2 bell pepper, diced
- 2 tbsp olive oil
- 1 tbsp lemon juice
- Salt and pepper to taste

Instructions:

• In a large bowl, combine cooked quinoa, mixed greens, cucumber, and bell pepper.

• Top with sliced grilled chicken.

• In a small bowl, whisk together olive oil, lemon juice, salt, and pepper. Drizzle over the salad and toss to combine.

2. *Turkey and Lettuce Wraps:*

Ingredients:

- 1 cup cooked turkey, shredded or sliced
- Large lettuce leaves (e.g., romaine or butter lettuce)
- 1/2 carrot, grated
- 1/2 cucumber, sliced
- 1 tbsp mayonnaise (check for low-FODMAP ingredients)
- Salt and pepper to taste

Instructions:

- Spread mayonnaise on the lettuce leaves.
- Layer turkey, grated carrot, and cucumber on top.
- Season with salt and pepper, then roll up the lettuce leaves to create wraps.

3. Lentil Soup:

Ingredients:

- 1 cup lentils (cooked, check for low-FODMAP)
- 1 carrot, diced
- 1 celery stalk, diced
- 1 can diced tomatoes (check for low-FODMAP)
- 4 cups low-sodium vegetable broth
- 1 tsp olive oil

- Salt and pepper to taste

Instructions:

- In a pot, heat olive oil over medium heat. Add carrot and celery, sautéing until soft.
- Add cooked lentils, diced tomatoes, and vegetable broth. Bring to a boil.
- Reduce heat and simmer for about 20-30 minutes. Season with salt and pepper.

4. Grilled Vegetable Salad:

Ingredients:

- 1 zucchini, sliced
- 1 bell pepper, sliced
- 1 cup cherry tomatoes
- 2 tbsp olive oil
- Salt and pepper to taste

- 2 cups mixed greens
- Balsamic vinegar for dressing

Instructions:

- Preheat grill or grill pan.
- Toss zucchini, bell pepper, and cherry tomatoes in olive oil, salt, and pepper.
- Grill vegetables until tender and slightly charred.
- In a bowl, combine grilled vegetables with mixed greens. Drizzle with balsamic vinegar and toss to combine.

5. Rice and Shrimp Bowl:

Ingredients:

- 1 cup cooked white rice
- 1 cup shrimp, peeled and deveined

- 1 tsp garlic-infused oil (for flavor, without FODMAPs)
- 1/2 bell pepper, sliced
- Salt and pepper to taste
- Fresh cilantro for garnish

Instructions:

- In a pan, heat garlic-infused oil over medium heat. Add shrimp and cook until pink.
- Add sliced bell pepper and cook for a few more minutes until tender.
- Serve shrimp and bell pepper over cooked rice, garnished with fresh cilantro.
- Feel free to adjust ingredients based on your tastes and dietary needs!

Dinner Recipes

Here are some delicious and simple low-FODMAP dinner recipes:

1. *Baked Salmon with Quinoa and Steamed Zucchini:*

Ingredients:

- 2 salmon fillets
- 1 cup quinoa
- 2 zucchinis, sliced
- 2 tbsp olive oil
- 1 lemon, sliced
- Salt and pepper to taste
- Fresh dill for garnish

Instructions:

- Preheat the oven to 375°F (190°C).
- Place salmon fillets on a baking sheet, drizzle with olive oil, and

season with salt, pepper, and lemon slices. Bake for 15-20 minutes, until cooked through.

- Cook quinoa according to package instructions.
- Steam zucchini slices until tender.
- Serve salmon over quinoa with steamed zucchini on the side, garnished with fresh dill.

2. *Grilled Chicken with Roasted Vegetables:*

Ingredients:

- 2 chicken breasts
- 1 red bell pepper, sliced
- 1 zucchini, sliced
- 1 eggplant, sliced
- 2 tbsp olive oil
- 1 tsp dried oregano
- Salt and pepper to taste

Instructions:

- Preheat grill or grill pan.
- Drizzle chicken breasts with olive oil, and season with salt, pepper, and oregano.
- Grill chicken until cooked through, about 6-7 minutes per side.
- Meanwhile, preheat oven to 400°F (200°C). Toss bell pepper, zucchini, and eggplant with olive oil, salt, and pepper. Spread on a baking sheet and roast for 20-25 minutes.
- Serve grilled chicken with roasted vegetables.

3. Beef Stir-Fry with Broccoli and Bell Peppers

Ingredients:

- 1 lb (450g) beef strips

- 1 head broccoli, cut into florets

- 1 red bell pepper, sliced

- 1 tbsp garlic-infused oil

- 2 tbsp soy sauce (gluten-free if needed)

- 1 tbsp rice vinegar

- 1 tsp sesame oil

- 1 tsp cornstarch mixed with 2 tbsp water

Instructions:

- Heat garlic-infused oil in a large skillet or wok over medium-high heat.

- Add beef strips and cook until browned. Remove from skillet and set aside.

- Add broccoli and bell pepper to the skillet, and stir-fry until tender.

- Return beef to the skillet. Add soy sauce, rice vinegar, and sesame oil. Stir to combine.
- Add the cornstarch mixture and cook until the sauce thickens.
- Serve over rice or quinoa.

4. Roasted Chicken with Mashed Potatoes and Green Beans:

Ingredients:

- 2 chicken thighs
- 2 tbsp olive oil
- 1 tsp dried thyme
- Salt and pepper to taste
- 4 potatoes, peeled and diced
- 1/4 cup lactose-free milk
- 1 tbsp butter
- 1 lb (450g) green beans, trimmed

Instructions:

- Preheat oven to 375°F (190°C).
- Place chicken thighs on a baking sheet, drizzle with olive oil, and season with thyme, salt, and pepper. Roast for 35-40 minutes, until cooked through.
- Boil potatoes until tender. Drain and mash with lactose-free milk and butter. Season with salt and pepper.
- Steam green beans until tender.
- Serve roasted chicken with mashed potatoes and green beans.

5. Shrimp and Rice Bowl:

Ingredients:

- 1 lb (450g) shrimp, peeled and deveined

- 2 cups cooked white rice
- 1 red bell pepper, sliced
- 1 cup snap peas
- 2 tbsp garlic-infused oil
- 2 tbsp soy sauce (gluten-free if needed)
- 1 tbsp lime juice
- Fresh cilantro for garnish

Instructions:

- Heat garlic-infused oil in a large skillet over medium-high heat.
- Add shrimp and cook until pink and opaque. Remove from skillet and set aside.
- Add bell pepper and snap peas to the skillet, and stir-fry until tender.
- Return shrimp to the skillet, and add soy sauce and lime juice. Stir to combine.

- Serve over cooked rice, garnished with fresh cilantro.

Enjoy these low-FODMAP dinner recipes! Feel free to adjust portions and ingredients according to your taste and dietary needs.

Snacks & Dessert Recipes

Here are some delicious and simple low-FODMAP snack and dessert recipes:

Snacks

1. Cucumber and Carrot Sticks with Hummus:

Ingredients:

- 1 cucumber, sliced
- 2 carrots, sliced
- 1 cup low-FODMAP hummus (check for low-FODMAP

ingredients like garlic-infused oil instead of fresh garlic)

Instructions:

- Arrange cucumber and carrot sticks on a plate.
- Serve with a side of hummus for dipping.

2. Rice Cakes with Peanut Butter and Banana:

Ingredients:

- 2 rice cakes
- 2 tbsp natural peanut butter
- 1 banana, sliced

Instructions:

- Spread peanut butter evenly on each rice cake.
- Top with banana slices.

3. Lactose-Free Yogurt with Berries:

Ingredients:

- 1 cup lactose-free yogurt
- 1/2 cup blueberries or strawberries

Instructions:

- Spoon yogurt into a bowl.
- Top with berries.

4. Hard-Boiled Eggs:

Ingredients:

- 2 eggs

Instructions:

- Place eggs in a pot and cover with water.
- Bring to a boil, then reduce heat and simmer for 9-12 minutes.

- Drain and cool under cold running water. Peel and enjoy.

5. Almonds and Grapes:

Ingredients:

- 1/4 cup almonds (in moderation)
- 1 cup grapes

Instructions:

- Serve almonds and grapes together in a bowl for a balanced snack.

<u>Desserts:</u>

1. Chia Pudding:

Ingredients:

- 1/4 cup chia seeds
- 1 cup lactose-free milk (or almond milk)

- 1 tbsp maple syrup
- Fresh strawberries or kiwi for topping

Instructions:

- In a bowl or jar, combine chia seeds, lactose-free milk, and maple syrup.
- Stir well, then refrigerate for at least 4 hours or overnight.
- Serve topped with fresh fruit.

2. Banana Ice Cream:

Ingredients:

- 2 ripe bananas, sliced and frozen
- 1 tsp vanilla extract

Instructions:

• Place frozen banana slices and vanilla extract in a food processor or blender.

• Blend until smooth and creamy.

• Serve immediately or freeze for a firmer texture.

3. Strawberry Smoothie:

Ingredients:

- 1 cup lactose-free yogurt
- 1 cup fresh or frozen strawberries
- 1 tbsp maple syrup (optional)

Instructions:

- In a blender, combine lactose-free yogurt, strawberries, and maple syrup.
- Blend until smooth.
- Pour into a glass and enjoy.

4. Oatmeal Cookies:

Ingredients:

- 1 cup rolled oats
- 1/2 cup almond flour
- 1/2 tsp baking soda
- 1/4 cup coconut oil, melted
- 1/4 cup maple syrup
- 1 egg
- 1 tsp vanilla extract
- 1/2 cup dark chocolate chips (optional, check for low-FODMAP)

Instructions:

- Preheat oven to 350°F (175°C) and line a baking sheet with parchment paper.
- In a bowl, mix together oats, almond flour, and baking soda.

- In another bowl, whisk together melted coconut oil, maple syrup, egg, and vanilla extract.
- Combine wet and dry ingredients, then fold in chocolate chips.
- Drop spoonfuls of dough onto the baking sheet.
- Bake for 10-12 minutes, until golden brown. Cool on a wire rack.

5. Lactose-Free Chocolate Pudding:

Ingredients:

- 2 cups lactose-free milk
- 1/4 cup cornstarch
- 1/4 cup cocoa powder
- 1/4 cup maple syrup
- 1 tsp vanilla extract

Instructions:

- In a saucepan, whisk together cornstarch, cocoa powder, and maple syrup.
- Gradually add lactose-free milk, whisking constantly to avoid lumps.
- Cook over medium heat, stirring constantly, until the mixture thickens.
- Remove from heat and stir in vanilla extract.
- Pour into serving dishes and refrigerate until set.

Enjoy these low-FODMAP snacks and desserts, tailored to help manage IBS symptoms while satisfying your cravings!

CHAPTER FOUR
Cooking Tips For Sensitive Stomachs

Cooking for sensitive stomachs, especially for those with conditions like IBS, involves selecting ingredients and preparation methods that minimize digestive discomfort. Here are some tips to help you create meals that are gentle on the stomach:

Ingredient Selection:

• **Low-FODMAP Foods**: Choose foods that are low in fermentable carbohydrates (FODMAPs) to reduce bloating, gas, and discomfort.

• **Lean Proteins**: Opt for lean proteins such as chicken, turkey, fish, and tofu, which are easier to digest.

• **Cooked Vegetables**: Raw vegetables can be hard to digest, so lightly steaming, roasting, or boiling them can make them gentler on the stomach.

• **Lactose-Free Dairy**: Use lactose-free milk, yogurt, and cheese to avoid lactose intolerance symptoms.

• **Gluten-Free Grains**: Quinoa, rice, and gluten-free oats are good choices if gluten sensitivity is an issue.

• **Healthy Fats**: Use small amounts of healthy fats like olive oil and avoid heavy, fried, or greasy foods.

Cooking Techniques:

• **Slow Cooking**: Slow-cooked meals, such as soups and stews, break down fibers and make foods easier to digest.

• **Gentle Cooking Methods**: Steaming, poaching, and baking are preferable over frying or grilling at high temperatures, which can make foods harder to digest.

• **Pureeing**: Pureed foods like soups and smoothies can be easier on the stomach.

• **Small, Frequent Meals**: Eating smaller, more frequent meals can help prevent overwhelming the digestive system.

<u>**Seasoning and Flavoring:**</u>

• **Use Herbs and Spices Carefully**: Avoid spicy foods and use herbs like basil, oregano, and ginger, which can aid digestion.

• **Garlic and Onion Alternatives**: Use garlic-infused oil or the green parts of scallions and leeks for flavor without the digestive issues that whole garlic and onions can cause.

Preparation Tips:

• **Soak and Rinse Grains and Legumes**: Soaking grains and legumes before cooking can reduce their phytic acid content and make them easier to digest.

• **Peel and Seed Fruits and Vegetables**: Removing skins and seeds can reduce fiber content and make foods easier to digest.

• **Hydrate Well**: Drinking water throughout the day can help digestion. However, avoid large amounts of water with meals to prevent diluting stomach acids.

Specific Food Tips:

• **Avoid High-Fat Foods**: High-fat foods can slow down digestion and cause discomfort.

• **Limit High-Fiber Foods**: While fiber is important, too much can cause bloating and gas. Balance your intake with low-fiber foods.

• **Chew Thoroughly**: Chewing food thoroughly can help start the digestive process and make it easier on your stomach.

Meal Planning:

• **Plan Balanced Meals**: Include a mix of proteins, carbohydrates, and fats in each meal to support digestion.

• **Avoid Late-Night Eating**: Give your stomach time to digest before going to bed to prevent nighttime discomfort.

By following these tips, you can create meals that are both nutritious and gentle on sensitive stomachs.

Stress Management Techniques, Regular Exercise And Its Benefits

Managing stress and incorporating regular exercise are crucial for maintaining overall health and managing conditions like IBS. Here are some effective stress management techniques and the benefits of regular exercise:

Stress Management Techniques

1. Mindfulness and Meditation:

• **Practice Mindfulness**: Focus on the present moment through mindfulness exercises. Apps like Headspace or Calm can guide you through mindfulness practices.

• **Meditation**: Spend a few minutes each day in meditation to reduce stress and improve mental clarity.

2. Deep Breathing Exercises:

• **Breathing Techniques**: Practice deep breathing exercises like diaphragmatic breathing or the 4-7-8 technique to activate the body's relaxation response.

• **Regular Practice**: Incorporate breathing exercises into your daily routine, especially during stressful moments.

3. Progressive Muscle Relaxation:

• **Technique**: Tense and then slowly release each muscle group in your body, starting from your toes and working up to your head.

• **Benefits**: Helps reduce physical tension and promote relaxation.

4. Yoga and Tai Chi:

• **Yoga**: Engage in yoga to combine physical movement, breathing, and meditation for stress relief and improved flexibility.

• **Tai Chi**: Practice Tai Chi for gentle, flowing movements that help reduce stress and improve balance.

5. Journaling:

- **Write It Down**: Keep a journal to express your thoughts and emotions. Writing about your experiences can help you process stress and identify stressors.

- **Gratitude Journaling**: Focus on positive aspects of your life by writing down things you are grateful for each day.

6. Time Management:

- **Prioritize Tasks**: Break tasks into manageable chunks and prioritize them to avoid feeling overwhelmed.

- **Set Realistic Goals**: Set achievable goals to maintain a sense of accomplishment and reduce stress.

7. Engage in Hobbies:

• **Find Joy**: Spend time on activities you enjoy, such as reading, painting, or gardening, to distract from stress and enhance your mood.

• **Social Interaction**: Engage in social activities and maintain connections with friends and family for support.

Regular Exercise and Its Benefits:

1. Types of Exercise:

• **Cardiovascular Exercise**: Activities like walking, running, cycling, or swimming improve heart health and boost endorphins.

• **Strength Training**: Incorporate weight lifting or resistance exercises to build muscle strength and improve metabolism.

- **Flexibility and Balance**: Yoga, Pilates, and stretching exercises enhance flexibility and balance, reducing the risk of injury.

2. Benefits of Regular Exercise:

- **Reduces Stress**: Exercise reduces the body's stress hormones, such as cortisol, and increases the production of endorphins, the body's natural mood lifters.

- **Improves Mood**: Regular physical activity can alleviate symptoms of depression and anxiety and improve overall mood.

- **Boosts Energy**: Exercise improves cardiovascular health, leading to increased energy levels and reduced fatigue.

• **Enhances Sleep**: Regular exercise can help you fall asleep faster and improve sleep quality, essential for overall health.

• **Supports Digestive Health**: Physical activity can stimulate the digestive tract and help manage symptoms of IBS, such as constipation and bloating.

• **Promotes Weight Management**: Helps maintain a healthy weight, reducing the risk of chronic diseases.

Incorporating Exercise into Your Routine:

• **Start Small**: Begin with short, manageable exercise sessions and gradually increase duration and intensity.

• **Find Enjoyable Activities**: Choose activities you enjoy to make exercise a fun and sustainable part of your routine.

• **Set Realistic Goals**: Establish achievable fitness goals to stay motivated and track your progress.

• **Mix It Up**: Vary your exercise routine to prevent boredom and work different muscle groups.

• **Stay Consistent**: Aim for at least 150 minutes of moderate-intensity exercise or 75 minutes of vigorous-intensity exercise per week, as recommended by health guidelines.

By incorporating stress management techniques and regular exercise into your daily life, you can enhance your overall well-being, manage IBS symptoms more effectively, and improve your quality of life.

Hydration is essential for maintaining overall health and well-being, especially for managing conditions like IBS. Here's why hydration is important and how to ensure you stay properly hydrated:

The Importance of Hydration

1. Aids Digestion:

• **Promotes Smooth Digestion**: Water helps break down food so that your body can absorb nutrients. It aids in the movement of food through the intestines.

• **Prevents Constipation**: Adequate water intake softens stools and promotes regular bowel movements, reducing the risk of constipation.

2. Regulates Body Temperature:

- **Thermoregulation**: Water helps maintain your body temperature through sweating and respiration. Proper hydration prevents overheating and supports normal body functions.

3. Supports Nutrient Transportation:

• **Nutrient Absorption**: Water is vital for dissolving vitamins, minerals, and other nutrients from your food and transporting them to different parts of your body.

4. Maintains Energy Levels:

• **Prevents Fatigue**: Dehydration can lead to fatigue and a decrease in physical and mental performance. Staying hydrated helps maintain energy levels throughout the day.

5. Enhances Physical Performance:

• **Exercise Efficiency**: Proper hydration is crucial for optimal physical performance. It helps maintain muscle function and prevent cramps and fatigue during exercise.

6. Supports Kidney Function:

• **Detoxification**: Water aids in the removal of waste products and toxins from the body through urine. Proper hydration supports kidney function and prevents kidney stones.

7. Improves Skin Health:

• **Hydrated Skin**: Adequate water intake helps maintain skin elasticity and appearance, preventing dryness and promoting a healthy complexion.

8. Boosts Cognitive Function:

• **Mental Clarity**: Dehydration can impair cognitive functions such as concentration, alertness, and short-term memory. Staying hydrated supports optimal brain function.

<u>Tips for Staying Hydrated</u>

1. Drink Plenty of Water:

• **Daily Intake**: Aim for at least 8 cups (64 ounces) of water a day, or more depending on your activity level, climate, and individual needs.

2. Incorporate Hydrating Foods:

• **Water-Rich Foods**: Include fruits and vegetables with high water content, such as cucumbers, watermelon, strawberries, and lettuce, in your diet.

3. Monitor Urine Color:

• **Hydration Indicator**: Use the color of your urine as a hydration indicator. Pale yellow urine usually indicates proper hydration, while darker urine suggests a need for more fluids.

4. Set Reminders:

• **Stay on Track**: Set reminders on your phone or use hydration tracking apps to prompt you to drink water regularly throughout the day.

5. Flavor Your Water:

• **Infusions**: Add natural flavors to your water, such as lemon, lime, cucumber, or mint, to make it more enjoyable to drink.

6. Carry a Water Bottle:

• **Convenience**: Keep a reusable water bottle with you at all times to make drinking water convenient and accessible.

7. Drink Before You're Thirsty:

• **Proactive Hydration**: Don't wait until you feel thirsty to drink water. Thirst is a sign that your body is already partially dehydrated.

8. Hydrate During Exercise:

• **Pre and Post-Workout**: Drink water before, during, and after exercise to replace fluids lost through sweat and maintain performance.

Hydration for IBS Management

1. Preventing Constipation:

• **Regularity**: Staying hydrated helps keep the digestive system functioning smoothly, preventing constipation, a common issue for those with IBS.

2. Managing Diarrhea:

• **Rehydration**: For those experiencing diarrhea, it's crucial to replace lost fluids to prevent dehydration.

3. Balancing Electrolytes:

• **Electrolyte Balance**: In cases of severe diarrhea or vomiting, consider electrolyte solutions to maintain a proper balance of minerals like sodium, potassium, and magnesium.

By prioritizing hydration and making it a consistent part of your daily routine, you can support overall health, enhance digestive function, and effectively manage symptoms of conditions like IBS.

CHAPTER FIVE

Herbal Remedies And Supplements

Herbal remedies and supplements can be helpful in managing symptoms of IBS and promoting overall digestive health. However, it's important to use them cautiously and consult with a healthcare provider before starting any new supplement regimen. Here are some commonly recommended herbal remedies and supplements for IBS:

Herbal Remedies

1. Peppermint Oil:

• **Benefits**: Peppermint oil has antispasmodic properties that can help relax the muscles of the gastrointestinal tract, reducing symptoms like bloating, gas, and abdominal pain.

- **Usage**: Enteric-coated capsules are often recommended to ensure the oil reaches the intestines without causing heartburn or irritation.

2. Ginger:

- **Benefits**: Ginger can help reduce nausea, improve digestion, and alleviate stomach discomfort. It has anti-inflammatory and motility-enhancing effects.

- **Usage**: Fresh ginger tea, ginger capsules, or adding ginger to meals can be effective.

3. Chamomile:

- **Benefits**: Chamomile has anti-inflammatory and calming properties that can help soothe the digestive tract and reduce symptoms like cramping and gas.

• **Usage**: Chamomile tea is a common way to consume this herb.

4. Turmeric:

• **Benefits**: Turmeric contains curcumin, which has anti-inflammatory properties that may help reduce gut inflammation and improve symptoms.

• **Usage**: Turmeric supplements or adding turmeric to meals can be beneficial. Pair with black pepper to enhance absorption.

5. Fennel:

• **Benefits**: Fennel can help reduce bloating and gas due to its carminative properties. It also helps in relaxing the muscles of the gastrointestinal tract.

• **Usage**: Fennel tea or chewing fennel seeds after meals can be helpful.

1. Probiotics:

• **Benefits**: Probiotics can help balance the gut microbiota, potentially reducing IBS symptoms like bloating, gas, and irregular bowel movements.

• **Types**: Strains such as Bifidobacterium infantis, Lactobacillus plantarum, and Saccharomyces boulardii are commonly recommended for IBS.

2. Fiber Supplements:

• **Benefits**: Soluble fiber supplements like psyllium can help regulate bowel movements and improve stool consistency.

- **Usage**: Gradually introduce fiber supplements to avoid exacerbating symptoms like gas and bloating.

3. Digestive Enzymes:

- **Benefits**: Digestive enzyme supplements can help break down food more effectively, reducing symptoms of indigestion, gas, and bloating.

- **Usage**: Take digestive enzymes with meals, especially those containing proteins, fats, and complex carbohydrates.

4. Vitamin D:

- **Benefits**: Vitamin D deficiency has been linked to IBS. Supplementing with vitamin D can help improve overall gut health and reduce symptoms.

- **Usage**: Consult with a healthcare provider for appropriate dosage based on your vitamin D levels.

5. Magnesium:

- **Benefits**: Magnesium can help relax the muscles of the gastrointestinal tract and alleviate constipation.

- **Usage**: Magnesium citrate is often recommended for its mild laxative effect.

Tips for Using Herbal Remedies and Supplements:

- **Consult a Healthcare Provider**: Before starting any new supplement or herbal remedy, talk to your healthcare provider to ensure it's safe and appropriate for your condition.

- **Start Slowly**: Introduce one new remedy or supplement at a time to monitor its effects and avoid overwhelming your system.

- **Monitor Symptoms**: Keep track of your symptoms to assess the effectiveness of the herbal remedy or supplement.

- **Quality Matters**: Choose high-quality supplements and herbal products from reputable sources to ensure safety and efficacy.

- **Avoid Interactions**: Be aware of potential interactions between supplements, herbal remedies, and medications you may be taking.

By carefully selecting and using herbal remedies and supplements, you can support your digestive health and manage IBS symptoms more effectively.

Dining out and traveling with IBS can be challenging, but with careful planning and awareness, you can manage your symptoms and enjoy your experiences. Here are some tips to help you navigate dining out and traveling while managing IBS:

Tips for Dining Out

1. Choose the Right Restaurant:

• **Research**: Look for restaurants that offer menu options catering to dietary restrictions, such as gluten-free, lactose-free, or low-FODMAP dishes.

• **Call Ahead**: Contact the restaurant to inquire about their menu and whether they can accommodate your dietary needs.

2. Review the Menu in Advance:

• **Online Menus**: Many restaurants have their menus available online. Review them beforehand to identify safe choices.

• **Ask Questions**: Don't hesitate to ask your server about ingredients, cooking methods, and potential substitutions.

3. Make Specific Requests:

• **Modify Dishes**: Request modifications to dishes, such as grilling instead of frying, or asking for sauces and dressings on the side.

• **Avoid Triggers**: Request the omission of common trigger ingredients like garlic, onions, and certain spices.

4. Portion Control:

• **Small Portions**: Order smaller portions or share dishes to avoid overeating, which can trigger symptoms.

• **Take Home Leftovers**: Don't feel pressured to finish large portions. Ask for a takeout container to bring leftovers home.

5. Safe Choices:

• **Simple Dishes**: Opt for simple, whole foods like grilled chicken, steamed vegetables, and plain rice or potatoes.

• **Avoid High-Fat and Fried Foods**: These can be harder to digest and may exacerbate symptoms.

6. Plan Your Meal Times:

• **Avoid Busy Hours**: Eating during quieter times can reduce stress and allow for more personalized attention from staff.

• **Eat Slowly**: Take your time to eat, chew thoroughly, and savor your meal to aid digestion.

Tips for Traveling with IBS

1. Plan Ahead:

• **Research Destinations**: Look for places with a variety of dining options that can accommodate your dietary needs.

• **Pack Snacks**: Bring safe, non-perishable snacks like rice cakes, low-FODMAP granola bars, nuts, and dried fruits.

2. Stay Hydrated:

• **Carry Water**: Keep a water bottle with you to stay hydrated, which helps with digestion and prevents constipation.

• **Avoid Dehydrating Beverages**: Limit intake of alcohol, caffeine, and sugary drinks.

3. Maintain Regular Eating Habits:

• **Consistent Meal Times**: Try to eat at regular intervals to maintain your digestive routine.

• **Balanced Meals**: Include a mix of proteins, carbohydrates, and fats to keep your energy levels stable.

4. Know Your Triggers:

• **Avoid Risky Foods**: Stick to foods you know are safe and avoid experimenting with new, potentially trigger-inducing foods.

• **Communicate Needs**: Don't be afraid to explain your dietary restrictions to hotel or restaurant staff.

5. Medication and Supplements:

• **Bring Essentials**: Pack any necessary medications, probiotics, digestive enzymes, and supplements.

• **Travel-Friendly Packaging**: Use travel-sized containers and keep them in your carry-on for easy access.

6. Stress Management:

• **Relaxation Techniques**: Practice deep breathing, meditation, or yoga to manage stress, which can exacerbate IBS symptoms.

• **Flexible Itinerary**: Allow for downtime in your travel schedule to rest and avoid stress.

7. Emergency Plan:

• **Know Locations**: Familiarize yourself with the locations of restrooms along your travel route.

• **Local Cuisine Research**: Learn about the local cuisine and identify safe options before you arrive.

<u>**Tips for Specific Situations**</u>

Air Travel:

• **Pre-Order Special Meals**: Many airlines offer special meal options like gluten-free or low-FODMAP. Order these in advance.

• **Stay Active**: Move around the cabin during long flights to aid digestion and reduce bloating.

Road Trips:

• **Pack a Cooler**: Bring a cooler with safe foods and drinks.

• **Frequent Stops**: Plan for regular breaks to stretch and use restrooms.

International Travel:

• **Language Barriers**: Learn basic phrases in the local language to explain your dietary needs.

• **Safe Food Choices**: Stick to cooked foods and bottled water to avoid potential gastrointestinal issues.

By following these tips and preparing in advance, you can enjoy dining out and traveling while managing your IBS symptoms effectively.

Conclusion

Living with IBS can be challenging, but with the right strategies and lifestyle adjustments, you can effectively manage your symptoms and lead a fulfilling life.

A comprehensive strategy that encompasses stress management, dietary modifications, and consistent physical activity is necessary to effectively manage IBS. By comprehending the distinctive triggers and requirements of your body, you can implement proactive measures to alleviate symptoms and enhance your quality of life.

It is important to seek the advice of healthcare professionals in order to develop a management strategy that is most suitable for your individual needs. By exercising mindfulness and meticulous planning, it is possible to overcome the obstacles of IBS and sustain a healthy, well-rounded lifestyle.

THE END